Diabetes & Obesity —Diabesity

A Genetic Curse or an Eating Hazard —How to Unmake the Mistake

Ahdy Helmy, MD, FACP

associate professor of medicine,
endocrinology, and metabolism
Indiana University

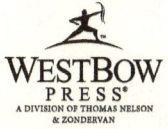

WESTBOW
PRESS®
A DIVISION OF THOMAS NELSON
& ZONDERVAN

WestBow Press books may be ordered through
booksellers or by contacting:

WestBow Press
A Division of Thomas Nelson & Zondervan
1663 Liberty Drive
Bloomington, IN 47403
www.westbowpress.com
1 (866) 928-1240

ISBN: 978-1-5127-8074-1 (sc)
ISBN: 978-1-5127-8075-8 (e)

Library of Congress Control Number: 2017904486

Print information available on the last page.

WestBow Press rev. date: 05/15/2017

Contents

Acknowledgments

First and foremost, I want to thank God almighty, the inventor and creator of this amazing machine, the human body, the fine tuning of which never ceases to amaze me. Its intricate structure and physiological accuracy cries out loudly in praise of the maker, emphatically stating, "I am not an accident, nor a product of million coincidences."

I pray He will grant me wisdom over intelligence and prudence in place of pride.

I then want to thank my gorgeous wife, Therese, for her love, support, and friendship. She is the love of my life and heaven's gift to me.

Next, I want to thank my two beautiful daughters, Sarah and Natalie, for their love and precious friendship.

Lastly, I want to dedicate this book to the memory of my dad, who lost his life in the battle with diabesity.

Knowledge is Power

This book is written to all people in all roles: parents, singles, adults, and adolescents.

My purpose is to equip them with knowledge delivered in a simple, yet meaningful way. My intent is to help them be of help to themselves, as well as to their loved ones. Their informed assistance will be of great help to us, the health care providers as we face Goliath, the giant that is "diabesity." A giant if left unchallenged is likely to swallow generations to come.

Introduction: "Why Bother"

We, as a society and as a world, are increasingly experiencing an epidemic of obesity. Obesity brings a whole cascade of consequences in the form of major health hazards, the foremost of which is diabetes. Diabetes is a disease of all organs, from our brain to our toes. This metabolic disease, with all its complications, is a burden to our health, finances, and abilities to do, achieve, and enjoy the gift of health.

How does this metabolic monster come into existence? Obesity is part of its origin. I'll merge the twin horns on the head of this hateful monster, diabetes and obesity, into one term and I'll call it *diabesity*.

The reason to come up with this relatively new term is that many of the factors leading to one or the other are common to the establishing of both. They coexist together in many individuals.

Though obesity may be easy to recognize in its extreme forms, many diabetics do not know they have it yet.

But "Why bother?" This is a great question. The simple answer is that there are 4,650 new cases of diabetes every 24 hours in the United States alone. Yes, you read the numbers right. There are more than 190 newly diagnosed diabetics in the United States every hour. And many of these cases are children, adolescents, and young adults.

The longer they have it, the more the complications they will develop. Let me just mention one stunning complication. In the United States alone, 180 diabetics lose a part or the whole of their leg every day, directly because of diabetes. Six of every ten who lose one of their legs to the disease will lose their lives within the next five years.

If that doesn't bother you, I do not know what will.

Chapter 1

Diabetes, the Silent Intruder

Diabetes, in its early stages of development, is asymptomatic. It sneaks up on us, uninvited, despite the fact that many of us may have some inner fears of diabetes, given our family history or sedentary lifestyle.

In the United States, type 2 Diabetes, which is the most prevalent type and, most often, has a partnership with obesity, takes about nine to twelve years on average to diagnose after it actually happens. Most of the new patients get diagnosed because of routine testing done for another problem, pregnancy, pre-employment, or because they wanted to try grandma's new glucometer.[1]

In many instances, the diabetics get diagnosed because they present with complications like peripheral neuropathy. That is the involvement of their tiny nerves resulting in persistent tingling and numbness of the toes, which keeps people, at times, from having a restful sleep. Some have gum disease, which is when they start losing their teeth at an earlier age. In this case, the dentist may the first to refer them for blood glucose testing. Persistent blurring of vision can also be one of those early complaints as the glucose in the blood gets higher and higher, it ends up pushing its' way into the lenses of the eyes. Those lenses get thirsty (almost, because of the higher osmolality of the sugar in them), and as they "drink" more water, they swell up, and this causes the vision to get blurry.

In these instances, usually the glucose is high enough to cause the individual to be feeling thirsty, which causes him or her to drink more, and urinate more frequently, larger volumes of urine.

Chapter 2

The Gatekeeper

Now before discussing what goes wrong, let me elaborate a bit about what goes right by expanding on the normal physiology or healthy body functioning that when it breaks, we have a problem or disease.

Sugar is a general term; what the body consumes and produces is *glucose*, as it is tracked and measured in the blood stream. It is the predominant sugar the body cells utilize and what the liver produces when fasting. It is an indispensable nutrition to the body's cells.

Our brain is an important example. Glucose is its most valuable form of nutrition, and it is the fuel that keeps it going around the clock. This vital and amazingly complex organ consumes about 50 percent of the daily total glucose consumed by the entire body. To be more precise, the brain, which is roughly about 3.5 kg in weight, consumes about 125 grams of glucose daily, while the rest of the body consumes another 125 grams of glucose.[2]

Now, what is responsible for transporting the glucose to the cells so that they can have their energy needs met? Insulin! Made specifically by specialized cells called beta cells in the pancreas, they cluster in the area of the pancreatic tail. Those beta cells collectively contribute to a small portion of total pancreatic volume. Beta cells are critical in providing this viable precious hormone that opens the gates to home deliver glucose to those body cells.[3] But do all cells need insulin, and when do we need this guy the most?

The brain, of all organs, can get the glucose into its cells in the absence of insulin. The brain's well-being is very critical, as it is the majestic headquarters of all operations. Any dependence on insulin could be very risky. The amazing intelligence that's behind this incredible body design cannot risk this. So while insulin may have some other, much less critical responsibilities in the brain, home delivery of glucose to the brain cells is not one of them. That's a blessing and a relief. Imagine diagnosing type 1 diabetes in a five-year-old child. By then, it would have been too late to save his brain if not for the independence of his brain from insulin for survival. In this case, the absence of the latter doesn't destroy the brain in those kids.[4]

Red blood cells can also get glucose into them without insulin's help. The brain and red blood cells are the biggest consumers for glucose during our fasting hours, like during our nighttime sleep.

While eating however, insulin is needed to facilitate the distribution of the glucose load building in our blood streams. It is very critical to dispose of the glucose building up in our blood, as fast as it builds up, and yet, it must be disposed of efficiently to where it is most needed.

During meals, the biggest glucose consumers are the muscles. The more toned and bulky the muscles are the more efficient and capable they are in the disposal process of the post-prandial (after a meal) glucose load.[5] In clinical trials, when regular exercise was combined with weight loss, it was more successful in preventing the progression of prediabetes to frank diabetes. One example is the Diabetes Prevention Program of North America and another is the Finnish Diabetes Prevention Study where 150 minutes of moderate activity with 7 percent weight loss were behind the prevention of prediabetes from progressing to frank diabetes in 58 of every 100 susceptible individuals.[6]

One of the developments of aging is the loss of muscle fibers as individuals get less active. The decline in the numbers of muscle fibers is a phenomenon called sarcopenia. It is one of the biggest risk factors for development of diabetes with aging.

Regular exercise and the preservation of those muscle fibers is an essential defensive mechanism against the development of diabetes. A confirmation of this critical issue is what we see among our adolescents and youth. More of them are succumbing to the metabolic syndrome and obesity and, eventually, type 2 Diabetes at a young age. It is the result of an unfortunate combination, the lack of exercise; hand in hand with more consumption of sugary drinks, most dangerously but not limited to regular sodas.[7]

As youths become more sedentary, they lose muscle mass. In addition, they consume too much sugar, creating an imbalance between a higher influx of glucose and calories in contrast to reduced disposition by muscles. This excess caloric influx and the increased conversion of the carbs into fats, will eventually lead to more fat getting stored and obesity to develop.

Obesity, to be specific, is an increase in fat stored in cells that, subsequently, expand in size and/or in numbers to meet the demands for storage.

Not all fat cells are created equal or are the same kind. Some are called visceral adipocytes. These tend to cluster around the gut in the middle section, are larger in size, more active, and have a higher tendency to recycle. Those visceral fat cells' location and bulk is highlighted by the waist circumference. It is sometimes called upper body obesity or midsection obesity.

Insulin, the physiological gatekeeper regulates the influx of glucose the nutrient into fat and muscle cells, as well as other body organs. It also preserves the body fat mass intact.

Chapter 3

Physiology, the Way It Was Meant to Be

Now, before diving into the concept of what it means to have so many fat cells, it should be explained that both visceral and subcutaneous fat cells are known as adipocytes from medical terminology standpoint. Ideally, there should be fewer fat cells, and they should all be working efficiently. These fat cells need insulin to keep them intact. The body provides insulin to prevent them from lipolysis, which is the breakdown of the fat load (triglycerides) into glycerol and fatty acids.[8] Simply put, insulin helps those cells to do their job as storage sites, and to keep their inventory of fat.

While in the fasting state, we do not need insulin to push the glucose into our brain cells. We do need some insulin to suppress lipolysis (to keep our fat stores from melting down). I always tell my students and medical residents that one of the reasons overweight and obese individuals have a hard time losing weight is because every time they accumulate fat, the body will generate enough insulin to protect it and preserve it. This is the body defense for survival; it is a physiological response. As we accumulate more fat, more insulin is needed to protect against lipolysis, and the cycle goes on, and what starts as physiology goes on to pathology. The longer the duration of obesity and the degree of obesity, the more insulin is produced. This insulin, needed to protect the fat, is required constantly and not only briefly during and immediately after meals.

Simply said, instead of the ideal scenario, where the pancreatic beta cells are working three or four times every day to handle meals, with obesity they are working multiple shifts and overtime, day and night to suppress lipolysis, to protect fat stores in addition to handling meals. They are at risk for burnout.

As if that's not enough, there is one more hurdle to consider. The adipocytes, or the fat cells in the midsection, called visceral adipocytes, tend to be larger and are heavily supplied with special receptors called adrenergic receptors. Those receptors are very sensitive to sympathetic stimulation, or, in simple terms, to the adrenaline, making them more ready for lipolysis or breakdown. The visceral fat is mainly designed for support of the organs, a cushion provided as a friendly supportive bed for the internal organs. They are not meant to be storage sites, and fat accumulation in them, represents a morbid build up.

It is as morbid as the abnormal deposition of fat and cholesterol in the human arteries, a place where under healthy conditions, should never have been a place for fat to accumulate.

As fat start to pour into those visceral adipocytes, they have a limited ability to increase in number, so they end expanding in size.

Quickly their size becomes too big for their mitochondria. The mitochondria for the cells are like the lungs for humans. They are essential to survive. As those adipocytes outpace in their growth the mitochondrial mass, they become unhealthy, in simple terms, sick.

Those sick visceral adipocytes develop a low grade inflammatory state as a result, and produce many inflammation-boosting factors that are very harmful to the body in general and offer more resistance to the insulin action in particular.[9] They also are inherently more prone to break down their triglyceride load. They need much more insulin to suppress them and keep them calm in comparison to what is required to keep the other subcutaneous adipocytes suppressed. Those subcutaneous (under our skin) adipocytes are generally called metabolic sinks. They are the naturally designed closets where surplus calories are stored as fat. That is separate from the midsection of our body where visceral adipocytes tend to reside, and where fat is not supposed to be diverted for storage.

Men tend to accumulate 20 percent of their extra fat in their mid-section while women tend to store 6 percent of their extra fat in their midsection. This upper body obesity (i.e., apple shape) is also called androgenic (given that it is male type). Compared to lower (or pear-shaped) obesity, it is the one that requires more insulin to preserve and attend to because of its' constituents, the visceral adipocytes.[10]

Again, remember this mid-section obesity, is not just fat accumulating in the waist line area, but is a hot bed of inflammation, a kitchen for an inflammatory soup, ready to dissipate its harmful ingredients throughout the circulation to the different organs, and body systems, including arteries, those carrying blood to our vital organs, like the brain, the heart and kidneys to mention few.

Some of the experts in the field describe this conglomeration of inflamed, sick adipocytes in the mid-section as the Sick Fat Syndrome.

Ideally, if our fat stores are kept to the minimum, we are in need for insulin to be released with the meals almost exclusively. Then it mostly disappears, in between meals, when it is not or minimally needed.

The body cells are designed to see and

respond to insulin intermittently with meals and thus maintain their sensitivity to insulin when it comes on board.

However, if insulin is called upon around the clock to keep fat stores from breaking down, in addition to being there with meals, the body cells get more and more used to the presence of insulin around the clock and gradually become desensitized to this valuable hormone.

This process is called insulin resistance, where insulin loses its effectiveness. In this instance, individuals need more insulin to provide the same effect that used to be achieved with less. Insulin resistance, unfortunately, is becoming more of an issue in our societies. This generally stems from higher caloric intake. This is, to a large extent, from carbohydrates, particularly simple sugars and gigantic sizes of fast food meals and snacks. The result is adipocytes storing more of what's not being spent. We are adopting a lifestyle as a society where we are spending lesser calories, as we exercise less and become more sedentary.

Sadly, that is happening even among individuals who are supposed to be the most active age groups: children and adolescents. This is in part secondary to electronics and video games that replaced physical activity, the mainstay to building muscles. More muscles would increase calorie spending, they are the power houses that turn energy loads into physical action and more muscles. A healthy cycle, likely would spare us from gaining more of, the specifically larger adipocytes. Consequently, would reduce the need for more insulin. Muscle building and an active lifestyle are key factors in keeping us insulin sensitive, and thus keeping insulin requirements to the minimum.[11]

Chapter 4

More Sound Physiology

It is remarkable to observe the body's ability to sustain harmony and balance, satisfying the constant need of glucose by the brain and the rest of the body, as it maintains a supply of it at all times. Whether, the individual is in the middle of a meal or fasting overnight.

In the fasting state, the liver, and to much less extent, the kidneys, are cranking glucose at a rate of 2mg/kg of body weight per minute at minimum and can be cranked up further as the needs dictate. If someone decides before breakfast, for example, to go and jog for six miles, the generation of glucose pouring into his or her bloodstream is crucial in keeping the plasma glucose from plunging in response to a high demand in the absence of food intake.[12]

In lay terms, the liver is a *giver* in the fasting state. It tunes into the existing demands and matches it to keep the blood glucose steady. The liver is doing that in the absence of insulin and in the presence of another hormone: glucagon. Glucagon prods the liver to produce glucose, when we are fasting. The purpose is to keep the blood glucose levels steady when there is no food coming. This glucose is indispensable for the survival of many of our cells, specifically the brain and the blood cells. That is in addition to the needs of the contracting muscles in the previous scenario.

The glucagon comes from another type of cells in the pancreas, which is different from, but next door to the cells making insulin. The alpha cells make glucagon, and the beta cells make insulin. Those two hormones are opposite in action and also in their timing (i.e., when to come on or off). The incoming of insulin ensures the outgoing of the glucagon, and that happens in ideal scenarios when our physiology is working unhindered.[13]

When we eat, usually we consume about 50–100 grams of carbohydrates with every meal (our entire plasma glucose pool is about 5 grams). This means we can get overwhelmed with such a load even with a healthy and stellar pancreas. The key in making this work is the liver. The liver changes its role from a *giver* in the fasting state to a *taker* in the fed state. The liver, in the fed state, will skim 40–50 percent of the glucose load in the meal, keeping it to itself. That helps to keep glucose from getting out of control in the blood stream.

Insulin, opposite to what the glucagon does, will make the liver stop giving. Simply makes the liver "shuts up" from further pouring glucose, and it actually turns the liver around to become a taker. The insulin is being secreted by the pancreas, and thus enters the portal circulation (circulation between the gut and the liver) first to reach the liver. The liver then shuts down giving, and as the feeding continues, the blood glucose accumulates in the peripheral circulation.

Sequentially, then the insulin starts slowly reaching the peripheral circulation, after going through the liver. It takes more insulin building in the peripheral circulation before the muscles which are actually less sensitive to the insulin than the liver, to start picking and disposing of the glucose.

This physiologically critical time lag guarantees not to run into the risk of low blood glucose in case the liver shuts down, while the muscles start simultaneously to dispose of the glucose instantly, or in close proximity.

The liver's ability to switch from a giver to a taker role then back to a giver again, all depends on it being a healthy liver, appropriately responding to many sequential and intricate, complex neural (mediated by signals transmitted along our nerves from higher brain centers) and hormonal signals.

Inflamed livers, for example, from hepatitis C, as well as fatty livers (e.g., storing excess fat within, and being on the receiving end of some of the inflammatory ingredients of the inflammation soup coming from the visceral adipose tissue in the mid-section), tend to become confused, and thus become slow or unable to switch roles.

These patients tend to be more susceptible, to develop type 2 diabetes.

Switching roles appropriately also requires the liver to be both, insulin sensitive and glucagon sensitive. That is to say, fully responsive to either hormones when they come to the scene.[14]

Chapter 5

Behind the Scenes

What else happens behind the scenes as the body physiology displays its genius engineering?

As we see, smell, and taste food, the first wave of insulin comes on board within a few minutes and convinces the liver to stop pouring glucose since food has been detected. The insulin, while well known as a master player, is like a celebrity who cannot do a good job without the help of many co-players that make its life much easier.

Following the first wave of insulin, another group of hormones (co-players) come from our gastrointestinal (GI) tract. We call those hormones *incretins*, which is short for "intestinal secretion of insulin." They boost insulin secretion that is precisely and smartly geared to how much glucose is coming in, without over-reaction or under-reaction.[15]

Those incretins, which include GLP1 (a glucagon-like peptide) and others, also work on the appetite to help reach satiety (i.e., curbing appetite). They help the individual to feel satisfied by working on the brain. It is a healthy brakes system, inherently protective to avoid over-eating. If operating as designed, it is a life-saver. Just remember as will-full creatures, we can always over-rule this friendly safe-guard.

The incretins shut down the alpha cells in the pancreas, and make sure the glucagon has exited out of the picture. And that the liver is assuming the role of a taker, following the instructions of the insulin alone, and again in proportion to how much insulin has been produced. Insulin amount, under the micromanaging style of the incretins will be precisely dependent on how much food is being consumed.[16]

Next in line to follow is a hormone called *amylin*, which comes from the beta cells, the same cells that make insulin. Amylin follows incretins, shortly after, to emphasize a curbed appetite and that the liver has stopped giving. Amylin also begins to aid incretins in slowing down the stomach in the process of emptying the food. The rate of exit of the meal from the stomach, and subsequently, the rate of appearance of the glucose in the blood stream has to match the rate of it's own disposal (consumption) from the plasma. Working together, both incretins and amylin will precisely adjust the influx of fuel to match the rate of its efflux. Those entering are equal to those exiting, without stacking, thus establishing a near-steady blood glucose level that's intricately regulated and finely tuned, even though it might be a thanksgiving meal that is being consumed.[17]

Shortly after this, comes the second wave of insulin, peaking about 50 minutes to an hour after the meal starts. It comes on board when the stage has already been set by a great orchestra. It works on the bulk of the accumulating glucose that is usually peaking about an hour after the first bite. So insulin comes just in time to handle this peak, and the stage is well paved by his previous co-workers. It is an orchestra of many players, and insulin adds its own touch to a grand finale.

Who would have thought that while we bite into a sandwich or a slice of cheesecake that there is an entire operation with many skilled players each pitching in? Each has a precise role in taking care of the meal for the best timely result, carrying the intended nourishment to where it is much needed, in the best timing possible. Following the meal, the most actively robust recipients of the glucose load would be the skeletal muscle cells. That's why the more we have of those "kind-to-us" cells the more efficiently the glucose load gets disposed of, without an increase of blood glucose level above normal boundaries. Glucose levels rising above those limits, is what we term medically as *postprandial* (after food) *hyperglycemia*. It is the early hallmark of pre-diabetes, what is given the term at times, impaired glucose tolerance. Think about it, it is intolerance to big meals, noting that the pancreas is losing its grip. When the post-prandial blood glucose reaches or exceeds a certain mark, 200 mg/dl, to be precise, it is diabetes disguised. Few years later, glucose becomes elevated all the time, not just following meals.[18]

On one hand, it is no wonder athletes can

consume significant number of calories: they have the muscle bulk to consume it efficiently, with their blood glucose remaining within normal.

And on the other hand, sedentary, insulin-resistant individuals, while they may consume fewer calories than consumed by athletes, will find that their blood glucose is building up. In those with fewer muscles, blood glucose will be standing in line, waiting to get into the very few muscle cells they have. It becomes more difficult, as they have fewer insulin responsive muscle cells, and more insulin resistant fat cells.

Healthy muscle cells are inherently more responsive to insulin. Even at times, they are capable of chewing glucose via other mechanisms, independent of insulin. Particularly, when actively contracting as in the middle of exercise. They need much glucose, in a rush, they cannot wait for enough insulin. So they pull the glucose into the cells before the insulin arrives to the scene. And this is a unique characteristic of actively contracting skeletal muscle cells.

Sedentary individuals have fewer muscle cells, and even some of those few became targets for fat deposition. They are being the recipients of the fatty acids originating at a distance from visceral adipocytes. The visceral lipolysis and fat stores melt down, causing the fatty acids to shower among other organs, healthy muscle cells. Turning them into unhealthy muscle cells harboring fats in between their fibers, and like many other organs in a sedentary individual they become more and more resistant to insulin, more like fat store keepers than glucose consumers.

Subsequently, more insulin is being required to push glucose into those resistant cells.

In a vicious cycle, the more insulin constantly circulating around, the more those unhealthy muscle cells and resistant fat cells become desensitized to insulin. Be it the basal insulin that is present at all times as well as the extra insulin that's called upon during meals. This results in a very inefficient disposal system, a deviation from what has been physiologically intended. And in many individuals, this broken system eventually crashes, as we will see later on in the book.

Chapter 6

Deviation from the Norm

Now, what really goes wrong? I hinted briefly to the deviations from normal physiology. Now, I would like to elaborate and explain how the disease develops as our body tries to adapt, although, despite good intentions, this is a maladaptation to the premorbid (i.e., setting the stage to develop disease) habitual and environmental behaviors.

We'll start with insulin resistance, which I explained before. It develops as a result of excess caloric intake with suboptimal calorie expenditure. This necessitates more storage, and thus, more adipocytes, which requires more insulin to suppress lipolysis in an attempt to preserve fat stores.

What aggravates this condition is the decrease of muscle bulk, the result of lack of regular exercise and a sedentary lifestyle. This decrease in the population of muscle cells, the big spenders, shifts the body to a saving mode, causing it to create a surplus of adipocytes, and the body gets caught in a self-perpetuating cycle of making and preserving fat cells.

Paradoxically, fat cells and muscle cells go separate ways. The more muscle cells you have, the fewer fat cells there are. Now, this is not as simple, because other factors contribute.

One major factor is the familial factor. This is not the same as genetics (genetics play a role, but quite small).

There are definitely genetic disorders that can present as insulin resistance, but those are quite rare. They do not contribute significantly to this epidemic of insulin resistance and what we call metabolic syndrome.

The family influence is a much more common contributor. This begins relatively early in life. It is estimated that by the age of two years, one third of children in the United States are overweight or obese.[19]

What I mean by the term *familial* is how family habits contribute to the individual ingrained dietary and activity behaviors. One example is the family habits of exercise, or the lack thereof. Another example is the family habit of skipping meals, especially breakfast. This gives the body a sense of insecurity, after many hours of fasting. Driving the body to store and hoard, thinking there must be a famine out there. That causes the body to slow down its own metabolism, a commonsense adjustment to skipping meals; a self-preservation instinct. The body stores to prepare itself for the worst. A third example is the family habit of eating big meals later in the day, where individuals are naturally hungry after skipping breakfast, lunch, or even both. Those big meals tend to be followed shortly after by sleep or prolonged periods of inactivity. All those are motives for the body to store and not to spend. Conclusively, the family is influential in establishing the eating and feeding habits of its members, starting quite early in life.

Storage and hoarding by the body becomes the dominant theme in absence of exercise and thus deficiency of muscle cells. Muscle cells can neutralize this tendency to store, since they are inherently known for big spending (burning fuel) and enhancing metabolism.

Insulin resistance means the job that used to be done by one unit of insulin cannot be satisfactorily performed. This means that two units, and with time, three, four units, and so forth, are needed to do the job that used to be done by one unit. Simply put, insulin resistance begets more insulin resistance.

The poor pancreas (the beta cells, the insulin makers, I mean), is now required to work day and night, to meet the ever increasing demands. The pancreas has to provide extra amounts of insulin to preserve those ballooning, stuffed fat cells, and to keep them from lipolysis.

As if, that is not enough, more insulin is also needed to dispose of the constant influx and rising glucose, as it is stacking in the blood stream. The reason is, that glucose is not being snatched quickly enough into the increasingly insulin hostile body cells. Those cells are resistant to the insulin action.

The pancreas is getting frustrated and stretched thin to the maximum to keep the job done, and the blood glucose level under control. Maximal pancreatic capability will vary from one individual to the other, meaning that, if the frustration of a stretched-thin pancreas is coupled with a family history of diabetes, the pancreas will end up crashing.

In simple words, it cannot keep up with those increasing demands; it cannot keep fat cells happy and suppressed, abstaining from breaking their triglyceride load into the loose cannons called fatty acids. While still, disposing of the glucose building up in the blood, efficiently. The pancreas failure means one outcome, glucose levels will start to rise up in the blood, and diabetes mellitus develops.

That is why type 2 diabetes, which is the more prevalent form of diabetes (more than 95 percent of all diabetic patients belong to this type) is often described as the disease of fatness, fitness, and family.

As the pancreas fails, this failure takes place initially after meals first, as they constitute the biggest challenge. That is to say, the pancreas can still keep the blood sugars at bay in the fasting state. But after meals, specifically larger ones, when stressed out and challenged with an overload of a carbohydrate rich meal while stretched thin as previously mentioned, it fails, as it gets overwhelmed, and it crashes hitting the floor with a bang.

Many individuals will have diabetes for years before the blood glucose in the fasting state starts to rise into the diabetes cutoff range. Only then, the patients get the official diagnosis of diabetes, which is often many years later.

That is why, as I hinted earlier, the first presentation of type 2 diabetes can be one of its complications, which has been in the making for years, since, in the United States, we usually resort to check fasting blood glucose to make the diagnosis. That puts us as health care professionals, usually ten to twelve years behind, between diabetes actually happening and the patient being officially diagnosed as a diabetic.

Chapter 7

What If?

What if the Pancreas doesn't crash? Are we off the hook? Wishful thinking! You cannot tip the balance and get away with it. The excess amount of insulin that is being produced around the clock because of insulin resistance, even if the pancreas can keep cranking it, is non-physiological. This means it is not the norm for the human body, as it is not a part of normal functioning and design.

The excess insulin will overwhelm the kidneys. Those generally are not as insulin resistant as the other body organs, namely the fat depots and sedentary muscles. The insulin levels, being elevated around the clock, whether during the fasting or the fed state, will cause the kidneys to retain sodium, and the body will retain secondary to that excess water. It is the body's inherent defensive adaptation to keep the blood sodium stable and prevent it from rising, is to retain an equi-osmolar amount of water.

This will cause volume expansion. That is to say, within the same fixed capacity of blood vessels, we are retaining more water volume holding to the excessively retained sodium.

Another phenomenon is the increased sympathetic activity, triggered by the excess insulin, and its central effect on the brain.

This is an interesting paradoxical impact at the brain level. Some areas of the brain are resistant to the insulin effect in curbing the appetite, causing over-eating. Other areas, on the contrary, are still sensitive to the insulin augmenting effect on the sympathetic nervous brain centers.

Both, the volume expansion and the sympathetic system over-activity will create a scenario where more spastic and less flexible blood vessels are carrying an expanding volume. And that eventually will lead to a higher blood pressure or hypertension.

High Blood Pressure augments the process of atherosclerosis, and subsequently the risk for heart disease.[20] We see more patients with their high blood pressure developing earlier than their diabetes, and some will develop the high blood pressure without ever developing diabetes.

That makes hypertension, a more consistent feature of insulin resistance and what is known as the metabolic syndrome.[21]

What else will be retained by the kidneys in response to the non-physiological excess of insulin, resulting from this insulin resistant state? You will be surprised.

It is uric acid, which causes many insulin-resistant patients to develop gout, which results from those uric acid crystals landing in their joints.

As we read the history of medicine, gout was often described as the disease of kings, and for years, the thought was, the excess meat-eating habits of kings, and nobles is the logical explanation. However, that is not the most accurate explanation. If you think more about it, obesity was uncommon several hundred years ago, except in palaces, where there was plenty to eat, and where people led a far more sedentary lifestyle.

The kings and royals were overweight, or obese and insulin resistant, while the common, hardworking, manually laboring common people were not.

High levels of uric acid, and gout as a potential result, becomes another consequence of obesity, and insulin resistance.

Now as industrialization sets in and

sedentary life habits become more prevalent, the curse of excess insulin brings over what was once relegated to the kings: gout, a disease that is quite painful and has nothing royal about it. We see this phenomenon in many third world nations as they move from more manual labor communities to more industrialization. This is being observed more and more in India and china where Diabetes is expanding in epidemic proportions. And Gout is not far behind.

Chapter 8

Metabolic Syndrome

So what is the metabolic syndrome? The *syndrome* is the term given by health care professionals to describe the consistent clustering of certain characteristic unhealthy conditions. Metabolic syndrome is based, first and foremost, on the presence of insulin resistance. The cluster of those characteristics were initially grouped under the name syndrome X, because the morbidity and long term complications were not yet fully appreciated in the medical community. And as X usually stood for the unknown in algebra, it was initially the name chosen.

Then it became the dys-metabolic syndrome, reflecting the disturbance inflicted on normal metabolism, and the hormonal harmony of the metabolic processes. Finally, a more simple terminology, the metabolic syndrome became more popular. A clear definition, without ambiguity is the first step to understand better and combat the metabolic enemy.

For insulin resistance to develop, obesity is the culprit. Obesity takes either, a more generalized form including the midsection obesity, as we encounter more among Caucasians and African Americans, or the rather more localized midsection obesity, as we see in people of Asian, Mediterranean, and Arab ethnicity.[22]

Often, midsection obesity is identified as a big waist line or a big waist-to-hip ratio. Second, in the ranking of importance, comes the presence of high blood pressure or hypertension. The other feature of metabolic syndrome is generally dyslipidemia or an aberration of the blood fats or lipids. This entails not necessarily high cholesterol but rather, a high triglyceride level, what we call *hypertriglyceridemia*. This is typically associated with lower high-density lipoprotein or what is known as HDL or the good cholesterol.

I help my patients to remember (HDL) as the type of cholesterol that is, "*H*ighly *D*edicated to *L*ift off cholesterol from their arteries." Generally, HDL has many roles, but it is widely believed to play an anti-atherosclerosis role by shifting cholesterol away from the blood vessels back to the liver.[23] And in doing so, it prevents the bad cholesterol (LDL) from accumulating like sludge inside of the blood vessels. Naturally, an elevated blood pressure helps this accumulation to take place, compounding the risk, when they coexist.

The combination of high triglycerides

and a low HDL play a significant role in atherosclerosis. Recent evidence looks at a low HDL as a marker of harm, rather than a direct cause of that harm.

Many experts call this combination, *atherogenic dyslipidemia* (a major contributor to making our arteries rigid, as it is geared to trigger an accelerated form of atherosclerosis).

The triglycerides get to be transformed down to smaller lipid components that are capable, given their smaller size to enter our blood vessels, triggering inflammation, and thus initiating and augmenting atherosclerosis (i.e., rigidity of the arteries).

Now LDL, or bad cholesterol, is the main threat to our arteries. The major player in atherosclerosis, LDL comes in different sizes; for simplicity, it comes in a larger form LDL a, and in a smaller form, LDL b. While LDL is bad, LDL b is worse ("*B*ader," is what I tell my medical residents and students) because it is smaller. It can sneak easier into the interior of the walls of our arteries and expedite atherosclerosis. It also uniquely expresses a highly negative charge. That promotes its ability to stick more easily to the blood vessel wall proteoglycans, an important component of the arterial wall.[24]

Atherogenic (atherosclerosis promoting) dyslipidemia, (i.e., higher triglycerides and lower HDL) favors the shift of LDL from the larger size, which is LDL a type, to the smaller, denser particles and more harmful LDL b type. One expert put it plainly: "While you can measure LDL b particles in the lab, an easier and cheaper way is to measure your patient's waistline." The bigger, the waistline generally, the more are the numbers of the smaller denser LDL b particles, potentially clogging the blood vessels.

Now let me mention another criterion in the metabolic syndrome: hyperglycemia which means an elevated blood glucose or sugar in common terms. This other criterion will be the net result of the stressed out pancreas. A pancreas overstretched to deal with the insulin resistance, reaches a point when it can barely make it. That is when the blood glucose levels start to rise higher than normal, above 100 mg/dl fasting.

Although this is still lower than the level required to diagnose diabetes, as the cut off level for the diagnosis is equal or above 126mg/dl fasting, those levels that are above normal but below diabetic range, are being referred to as *impaired fasting glucose. Impaired glucose tolerance* is the term used, when two hours after the meal, the glucose levels are elevated to above the usual 130-140, but still below the 200 limit necessary to make the diagnosis of diabetes(that is only after meal, but returns back within normal limits when fasting).

Those two states are described in the medical community as a *pre-diabetic state.* The patients described above, are at a higher risk to develop frank diabetes. Although in some of those patients, glucose levels can be restored back to normal if serious lifestyle modifications take place. That is especially true as they lose the excess weight and specifically mobilize their midsection fat excess.[25]

Now those patients, who restore a normal or near normal glucose values adopting a better life style, while their pancreas is still lame, its reduced ability will be enough to maintain normal glucose levels, when faced with lesser insulin resistance.

Another group of those who have hyperglycemia would be the established diabetics who went through the insulin resistance, the pancreatic overstretching, and its eventual crash.

It is safe to say that patients with insulin resistance are diabetics in training. Sitting on this insulin resistant state long enough to stress the pancreas, will uncover in many seemingly healthy subjects the inherent weakness of the pancreas to cope with such high demands. In others, the pancreas is capable to continue flooding the blood and the body tissues with excess insulin, the tissues that are insulin resistant and those that are not that much resistant.

Now, let me go back to hypertri-glyceridemia and elaborate on its nature and development. With insulin resistance, the visceral adipocytes become especially insulin resistant over time and break down regardless of the excess insulin that was secreted to make them not do that in the first place. This causes a constant state of lipolysis, that while significant and steady, is in no way massive enough to get rid of them. (Sorry to bust your hopes.)

The visceral adipocytes triglyceride load, which is the stored form, breaks down into free fatty acids. Those free fatty acids pour into the circulation in our gut area where the bulk of blood goes through a section of our circulation called the portal circulation.

Portal circulation from the gut area pours into the liver, its major and first filtering station. Now all those free fatty acids will bombard the liver. This major influx of fatty acids will put the liver in self-defense mode. The liver will repackage those free fatty acids back into triglycerides and send them into the blood to save itself from being overloaded. The excess flux of triglycerides into our blood will cause hypertriglyceridemia to develop. Eventually, the liver gets overwhelmed, and the excess triglycerides override the packaging and sending-out processes. Basically the ability of the liver to produce Apo B, a special protein that bound those triglycerides-rich lipid particles together, to form VLDL (very low density lipoproteins) and send them out into the systemic circulation, crumbles under pressure.

The fats start to deposit in the liver, leading to what we call a fatty liver or "nonalcoholic fatty liver disease" to differentiate it from a similar scenario that develops in heavy alcoholics. Nonalcoholic fatty liver disease is, unfortunately, very common among metabolic syndrome patients.[26] Their livers are assaulted in a manner similar to what happens with chronic and heavy alcohol consumption.

Also, the constant streaming of fatty acids into the portal circulation, coming from the visceral adipocytes in the mid-section will stimulate the liver to make more fat (lipogenesis) and glucose (gluconeogenesis). And both will compound the problems of high glucose and high fat simultaneously.

Some of those fatty livers get chronically inflamed, and the condition can eventually progress to cirrhosis, requiring liver transplantation. This is alarming, even though only a small percentage of fatty livers do progress to this chronic inflammatory state, described in medical terms, as non-alcoholic steatohepatitis (NASH). It is a small percentage of cases. Still, a small percentage of the many millions of metabolic syndrome patients of all ages will translate into an overwhelming large number of liver disease victims.

In simple terms, those fatty acids, generated as a part of the bigger picture, which is the insulin resistant state, can cause as much damage as long-term, heavy alcohol consumption. The difference is that those non-alcoholic fatty livers may start "drinking" a lot earlier in life, so to speak.

In one disturbing statistic, the prevalence of metabolic syndrome is nine percent among our eighth graders in the United States.

Given, the estimated eighty million individuals with metabolic syndrome in America alone, that potentially can translate to an overwhelming number of cirrhotic livers. In fact, after the development of the hepatitis C cure, this type of fatty liver turning to cirrhosis will become the more prevalent cause of cirrhosis in the near future.

Now, with hypertriglyceridemia, those packaged triglycerides in our blood stream termed Very Low Density Lipoproteins (VLDL), will exchange with HDL, taking some of its cholesterol, and lending it some triglycerides instead, through a complex mechanism which causes the HDL to become lower and less efficient in lifting off the cholesterol load from the arteries.

The final picture is far from pretty. A conspiracy on the body health, including accelerated atherosclerosis of the blood vessels, livers turning fatty and more resistant to the role changing from glucose givers to takers and vice versa. Also the blood pressure being elevated, and a net outcome of more heart attacks, strokes, cirrhosis, and liver failure.

The triglycerides that break off from the fat cells in the midsection, will get eventually to the general circulation as free fatty acids, and like loose cannons, will end up in our muscles, where many of them get transformed to triglycerides and end up being stored as fat.

Those muscles ending up with excess fat depositing in between its fibers, will become less effective in picking up blood glucose. In simple terms, those fatty acids spread the curse by making the muscles more insulin resistant, meaning their contribution to the disposal of glucose becomes less and less, eventually losing their inherent advantage as efficient consumers of glucose.

By turning those muscle cells into insulin-resistant cells is to turn them against us; and in metabolic terms, making those friends less friendly.

Those free fatty acids—the loose cannons—are also very capable of inciting inflammation. They also end up in the same cells (the beta cells) that make insulin in the pancreas, setting them on fire. By this, I mean triggering inflammation within those cells. This is similar to the inflammation that sets in fatty livers, causing a chronic inflammatory state. The inflammation within the beta cells will cause a constant decline in their functional ability to provide insulin. The beta cells, as a result, get weaker, and while the demand for insulin is higher, the beta cells' ability to make insulin is in decline.

The beta cells eventually burn out, and we see our diabetics starting on one medication for their high blood sugar. Then, over the years, they need more and more medications, and still their blood glucose average is on the rise as their beta cells' ability to make insulin declines progressively over the course of the disease.

Those loose fatty acids end up settling in the heart muscle as well, and while all the implications are not fully understood, inflammation is likely playing a major role. Some experts suggest the term *cardiac steatosis* (fatty heart), for its resemblance to the liver steatosis (fatty liver). The result is a subtle but progressive decline in the heart muscle flexibility & contractility. In its extreme form, it leads to diastolic heart failure. Simply said, the heart fails to relax fully. The heart muscle becomes stiff, unyielding and that impairs its ability to pick up enough load of blood to pump forward.

Recent data, using advanced imaging techniques as multiple cuts CT scan, revealed a strong correlation between EAT (Epicardial adipose tissue) and non-alcoholic fatty Liver disease. EAT is the collection of adipocytes accumulating between the myocardium, or the heart muscle and the first layer of the pericardium, which is the visceral pericardium. The pericardium itself is a soft double sheet cover of the heart. That correlation points to a common mechanism, for boosting this type of abnormal fat deposition in two separate, but equally vital organs.

Going back to ground zero, those visceral, midsection fat cells are larger and sicker. They are simply a hotbed of low-grade inflammation. From that flaming crate, inflammatory mediators (messengers) will spread to the body organs, as well as to the blood vessels, spreading a low-grade, smoldering inflammation throughout the body.

What is significantly alarming, that it is a rather common scenario among millions who have this metabolic syndrome.

It is a metabolic form of global warming, with far-stretching health implications, the longer its metabolic flaming pathology continues.

One more point I want to make clear: I elaborated on the liver as a giver and a taker of glucose and on the mechanisms behind the development of non-alcoholic fatty livers. While the liver on one hand, has an inherently well designed mechanism in letting glucose in, that is regulated under physiological conditions.

High-fructose corn syrups used to sweeten regular sodas and other drinks, on the other hand, has its own mechanism of forcing its way in an unregulated manner. Consumption of high-fructose corn syrup can cause a fatty liver to develop in a much faster way. So, that's a major problem for regular consumers of high volume of soft drinks.

In more than one study, fatty liver developed in cohorts of young healthy volunteers consuming 40 ounces of regular soda daily, after only 6 months.

The major concern, that those same young age groups, are likely to survive long enough, to reap the consequences of fatty hearts and livers.

That is in addition, to the soft drinks contribution to the non-nutritional caloric excess boosting the obesity epidemic.[27]

Chapter 9

Disarming the Metabolic Bomb

Now, after dropping this ticking bomb in the reader's lap, is there any way to disarm this metabolic hazard? Reversing insulin resistance is the only hope. It entails reversing what has triggered the resistance in the first place by reducing the adipocytes load. This is done by losing the fat, especially the more evil, visceral fat that settles in the midsection.

At the same time, increasing and attaining more of those muscle cells, the power houses that burn more energy to drain fat stores and transform us to be bigger spenders of calories, is equally important.

Diet and Exercise go hand in hand, and while there are so many diets out there, some are better than others. I will stick with the broad principles. Diets that provide the same caloric restriction but differ in protein, carbohydrates, and fat content are equally effective in achieving weight loss, as per clinical studies. However, within the first six to twelve months after the start of a nutritional intervention, carbohydrates restriction (i.e., "low-carb diets," especially the ones that restrict refined carbohydrates like sweets), typically lowers triglycerides more than a low Fat diet that is higher in carbohydrates. And this tends to lead also to faster weight loss.

Again for emphasis, weight loss can be attained with lifestyle programs that provide about 500–750 calories per day energy deficit, or in other words, allocate approximately 1,200–1,500 kcal/day for women and 1500-1800 kcal/day for men, adjusted for the individual's baseline body weight, and activity level.

Although benefits may be seen with as little as 5 percent weight loss, especially for lowering high blood pressure, sustained weight loss of 7 percent or more is optimal to partially protect against the progression of a pre-diabetic stage to frank diabetes.[25]

Mild body weight loss (e.g., 3 kg) may decrease mean triglycerides by 15 mg/dl. A sustained weight loss of 5–8 kg may reduce mean LDL-C approximately 5 mg/dl and increase mean HDL-C levels up to 3 mg/dl. We can see here that the biggest impact of weight loss is on the triglycerides, while on other fat parameters to a lesser extent.[28]

Among patients who are overweight or obese, systematic reviews of randomized clinical trials suggest clinically meaningful changes in atherosclerotic cardiovascular disease risk factors with at least 3 percent reduction in body weight. And further improvements with greater weight loss.

The only way to lose weight is to spend more calories than you take in. The plan is to eat more frequently, but fewer bites each time, using smaller plates. Striving for three small meals and two or three healthy snacks is a good plan.

Fill up on vegetables, especially, the less starchy, lower carbs vegetables such as broccoli, cabbage, celery. Also leafy vegetables like spinach, lettuce, collards, and kale are richly nutritious, high in fibers, and vitamins like folate which is an especially useful vitamin for future moms.

Leafy greens also contain calcium, magnesium which improves insulin sensitivity, iron, vitamins A and C. They are also rich in short-chain fatty acids that are converted in the gut to vitamin K, a fat soluble vitamin essential for the normal blood clotting physiology.

Remember, vegetables that are high in potassium and lower in carbs, like Brussel sprouts, spinach, and tomatoes help in sparing the body cells from importing too much sodium, as it gives the cells the potassium that they need in a very natural and easy-to-take form.

Ideally, two thirds of the plate should be vegetables of different colors.

The processed meals we consume more of, whether lunch meat, deli, canned foods and even bread are loaded with sodium. The fruits and vegetables are the main source for potassium, and what we tend to use less of. The imbalance in the dietary preferences creates a need for the cells to meet their interior need for the potassium that they cannot get enough of. The body cells, and more specifically, those endothelial cells that line our arteries and arterioles, are generally hungry for potassium because of their relatively higher rate of turn over and constant renewal. Attempting to balance their electrolytes, the cells allow a small but a pathological traffic of sodium into the cells. This is followed by calcium minimal influx. The calcium ions habit is to follow sodium. This calcium shift, while minimal, is still sufficient to increase the tone of the vascular tree, contributing to a higher blood pressure.

The extra sodium in our diet and the lack of potassium from fresh fruits and vegetables is believed to be one of the main reasons for the higher prevalence of high blood pressure in the West. The American Society of Hypertension stresses the importance of the balance between sodium and potassium in the diet; again, I mean natural sources of potassium like that found in fruits and vegetables, not from potassium supplements.

This has been shown in the DASH trial, (*D*ietary *A*pproach to *S*top *H*ypertension trial). This trial added more to our understanding of why high blood pressure is more prevalent in the Western world.

The DASH and Mediterranean diets (diets high in vegetables, fruits, legumes, lentils, nuts, fish, low-fat dairy, lean meats, and unsaturated oils) are both excellent approaches to protect our children from obesity, diabetes, and high blood pressure later in life. The earlier we start this, limiting salt while increasing intake of potassium-rich foods, will help reduce the chances of high blood pressure while arteries are still flexible, like those of our children. Of course, this is provided that there is no allergy to any of those dietary items.

Another disadvantage of a higher intake of salt (Sodium) besides the high blood pressure is its ability to drive more calcium into the urine. Excess sodium in, is excess sodium out through the kidneys and in the urine. As sodium gets kicked into the urine, calcium tends to follow. This will have a negative impact on bone health on the long run. That was shown in the Framingham study subjects, where women consuming high sodium had two folds increase in the risk of osteoporosis or bone fragility.

Getting proteins from grains and nuts like almonds will help to sustain and satisfy the body longer, without causing it to feel hungry sooner, and thus give in to unhealthy snacks.

These types of proteins can also replace animal proteins, which are inherently higher in saturated fat. Grains and nuts also provide fibers. Those can lower the cholesterol by displacing it away from absorption portals.

Fibers also regulate bowel movements. They have a tendency to drink water, and thus become bulking agents that enhance the colonic motility. More Colonic motility lowers the need for the colon to contract trying to squeeze out its' contents. That will protect the colon from an increased intra-colonic pressure and thus diverticulosis, a disease more common in people utilizing low fiber, highly refined Western diets.

In addition to vegetables, nuts and at least two to three servings of fruit daily, oats, legumes, and barley are rich sources of soluble fibers.

Generally, most professional organizations recommend viscous fibers at 20–30 gm/day.

Fibers, in addition are slowly digested and absorbed, causing a longer sense of fullness. They also tend to produce a lower blood glucose rise after a meal, what is technically termed Post Prandial Peak (PPP) of blood glucose. Fibers also tend to rein in other macro-nutrients consumed with them leading to a lower glycemic index (GI) overall, for the consumed meal.

The glycemic Index is a concept developed in the eighties, comparing the magnitude and speed of elevation in blood glucose following the consumption of different food items with pure glucose which has the glycemic index of 100 as a reference point.

The higher the glycemic index, the more robust is the expected response from the pancreas in terms of insulin secretion. The theory is, the more times the pancreas is pushed to the maximum, the more it is likely to burn out so to speak, specifically, if it is being born with limited capabilities, or is living in a pre-diabetic state.

Non-starchy vegetables like broccoli, and cabbage, whole grains, legumes, and lower carbohydrate fruits tend to have lower glycemic index. In the fruits, berries and cherries will have GI in the 20 range, while watermelon has a GI of 72, banana, cantaloupe in between with a GI of 50-60 range, again the more ripe the fruit, the more will be the GI.

Lentils and chickpeas will have a GI of

25-30. Carrots have a GI of 72. Highly refined carbohydrates can cause a fast and furious elevation in the blood glucose. The pretzels have a GI of 83, higher than that of skittles which is around 70.

Moderate use of good fats, rich in unsaturated fatty acids is also advisable to achieve a balanced healthy diet. Healthy oils like olive oil, around two table spoons daily, preferably more than half of this quantity uncooked, for instance as a salad dressing, is also recommended.

A good source of fat is nuts, as their fatty acids are monounsaturated and polyunsaturated. Some nuts, like English walnuts, are rich in certain fatty acids, that the body can convert a small percentage of it into fish-like type of fat at the molecular level. That works well for those who do not like, and are not willing to try fish.

Speaking of fish, especially fatty fish, which is generally cold water fish like halibut, salmon, mackerel, and tuna, eating this type of fish provide our bodies with a healthier fat that tends to lower triglycerides. (As I listed earlier, high triglycerides are a common feature of the metabolic syndrome).

Fatty fish like Salmon, Halibut, and Tuna is also a good source of vitamin D, which is a fat soluble vitamin that tends to be stored in body fat. Vitamin D is an essential vitamin for many of the cellular operations. But most importantly, it is critical for the bone health.

Because vitamin D is formed within the skin after exposure to sunlight, it is commonly deficient in northern states where less ultraviolet rays of the right wavelength penetrate to reach the skin.

Just remember, frying fish is not the best way to get those benefits as you are adding additional, unwanted fat and calories to your fish. Preferably, broil, bake, or grill the fish.

While on the subjects of vitamins, I noticed with my patients, that vitamin B complex and specifically vitamin B6 helps to lower cravings for sweets among some individuals, a humble observation I noticed over my twenty plus years of clinical experience.

Additionally, fill up your glasses with water. Data suggest that juicy, hydrated muscles burn more calories than less hydrated muscle cells. It is also an excellent remedy to avoid cramps, often encountered in the elderly, who generally feel less thirsty. As we age, our osmolality regulating centers in the brain, which determine the viscosity of our plasma, get reset, and it takes a higher osmolality, that is to say more concentrated plasma to stimulate our thirst centers.[29]

Caffeinated beverages are not the same as water, either. Caffeine is a diuretic, causing the kidneys to make more urine, so that is not actually hydrating the muscles. Remember, caffeine also drives more calcium into the urine, and in losing calcium, subsequently that will be harming the bones. This will impact the skeleton health adversely in the long term.

There is nothing like drinking water to hydrate the contracting muscles and the entire body tissues. Water should be the preferred beverage, which again should be a healthy habit ingrained early on during early childhood years.

For individuals trying to lose weight, an 8-12 ounce glass of water before meals may go a long way.

Also switching a can of regular soda to a big glass of water cuts back 225 Kcal daily, that translates into 82,125 less calories a year, and as much more hydration.

There is also credible data to suggest that even calorie-free, caffeine-free but artificially sweetened beverages make the brain less aware of the point at which the stomach is getting full. It almost interferes with the clarity of perception of the satiety centers. Those centers, sense fullness, and signal to prompt the brain to stop eating. Generally, individuals can help this awareness also by eating slower, chewing better, and taking the time to enjoy their food.

There are also data from small studies showing an increased absorption of carbohydrates from meals that follow the consumption of beverages sweetened with artificial sweeteners. They can also potentially slow the body metabolism. It is ironic, that while consuming sugar-substitutes is an attempt to reduce calories, this alternative may lead to an unintended surplus of calories being collected and stored in.

Exercise is equally important to diet, so exercise regularly rather than vigorously, and the advice is to encourage choosing an activity that the individual enjoys. That will ensure that, in all likelihood, he or she will keep doing it over the long term. My advice to my patients is to be consistent, remain focused, and be persistent.

Human bodies are smart, and in response to regular exercise and loosing calories, the body lose visceral fat first. The body perceives it is the most harmful, and that those fat cells are not supposed to be there in the first place.

So I tell my patients who diet and exercise but do not see their weight dropping on the scale, "Your muscles that you built are heavier than the fat cells; however, you'll notice your waistlines are getting smaller, despite an unchanging scale weight number."

Eventually, however, as more muscles get built, the weight will start to drop to the healthier range. But more importantly, there will be a healthy balance of muscles and fat in a relevantly healthy distribution.

Losing the weight slowly, while building skeletal muscles, keeps the extra weight off, and avoid the common rebound of the lost pounds. Those muscles, the power houses have a sustained, inherently higher basal metabolic rate. In simple terms, they burn more calories, keeping the body more in the spending mode, sparing less to hoard.

There are plenty of exercise studies showing that short-term exercise, especially aerobic activity, has a significant impact on triglycerides, especially those rising in our blood following a meal. It lowers this type of fat by up to 50 percent, which may persist for as long as forty-eight hours after the dynamic (aerobic) exercise training.[28] A very good reason to exercise regularly, or at least not allowing more than two days to elapse between exercise sessions.

We need to be consistent rather than impulsive. Triglycerides are the most common lipid abnormality we encounter with the metabolic syndrome, but also the most modifiable with healthy diet and exercise. At exercise training volumes of

1,200-2,200 kcal/week (e.g., fifteen to twenty miles per week of brisk walking or jogging), triglyceride levels may be reduced by 4–37 percent, HDL c levels increased by 2–8 percent, and LDL c levels ranging from no change (although likely a shift from the more harmful LDL b to the bigger in size and less harmful LDL a) up to a 7 percent reduction.[28]

Children should be encouraged to engage in at least sixty minutes of physical activity each day.

Recent evidence supports the fact, that all individuals, and especially those with diabetes, should be encouraged to reduce the amount of time spent being sedentary (e.g., working at a computer, watching TV). It is important to break up extended amounts of time (more than 30 minutes) spent sitting by briefly standing or walking, that is for the blood glucose benefits.[30]

Increasing unstructured physical activity

(incidental, non-exercise) like errands, household tasks, dog walking, or gardening increases daily energy expenditure, assists with weight loss, and with maintaining a healthy muscle vs adipose tissue distribution.

Even in brief (3-15 minutes) bouts, incidental activity is effective in acutely reducing the after meal spikes in blood sugars. It improves overall the degree of glucose control among pre-diabetics, as well as both type 1 and type 2 Diabetes patients.

Unstructured activity initially, can be a transition or a stepping stone, for those who are sedentary and unable or reluctant to participate in more structured exercise.

It is advisable, based on clinical data and expert opinions, that gradually and progressively overtime, adults over the age of eighteen years do 150 minutes every week of moderate intensity (e.g., power walking). Or 75 minutes of vigorous intensity aerobic physical activity (e.g., jogging) every week, or an equivalent combination of the two.

Children and adolescents, and more so those with type 1 or type 2 Diabetes should engage in 60 minutes /day or more of moderate or vigorous intensity aerobic activity. With vigorous, muscle-strengthening activities included at least 3 days every week.

Acutely, aerobic exercise increases the muscle uptake of glucose by about five folds, using an insulin-independent mechanism that continues to operate for up to two hours after the exercise has ended.

On the other hand the increase in the insulin-dependent glucose uptake (which means better insulin sensitivity) tends to continue for about a day after exercise durations of less than twenty minutes, and up to 2 days after longer exercise periods if the intensity of the exercise is elevated to near maximal. That is not to under-estimate low intensity aerobic exercise, which when lasting an hour or more can significantly enhance insulin action among obese subjects for up to twenty four hours.

Regular aerobic training increases the muscles insulin sensitivity in type 2 Diabetes patients and also among pre-diabetics, in proportion to the exercise volume.

Regular aerobic exercise may also prevent the development, or slow the progression of peripheral neuropathy, a common complication involving the nerves among diabetes patients both type 1 and type 2.

In one study even, the University of Utah type 2 diabetes study, they reported nerve fiber regeneration in patients engaged in an exercise program compared with loss of nerve fibers in those who only followed standard of care.

In addition, the guidelines suggest that adults do muscle- strengthening activities (resistance training) that involve all major muscle groups, two or more days (sessions) every week.[31]

Each session should consist of at least one set of five or more different resistance exercises involving the large muscle groups. Clinical trials have provided strong evidence for the glucose-lowering value of resistance training, especially in older adults with diabetes, using free weights or weight machines.[32]

Older adults are specially, at a higher risk for diabetes as I mentioned earlier in the book because of muscle loss. Muscle strength declines by about 15% every decade after the age of 50 years, and 30% after the age of 70 years.

Resistance training can cause 25-100% strength gain in those high risk groups. Also for older adults, especially with diabetes, flexibility and balance training are recommended 2-3 times every week. Yoga and tai chi may be included based on individual preferences. Many lower-body and core-strengthening exercises concomitantly improve balance.

Both aerobic and resistance muscle training, when done regularly increase the muscles capillary density, improving the blood perfusion to the contracting muscles. Rendering them more robust in carrying exercise longer, and in burning more calories efficiently to provide the best performance. It also increases the oxidative capacity, lipid metabolism, and insulin mediated signal proteins, that help insulin to work better within the muscle cells. Simply, improves insulin sensitivity.

Indirectly, and since organs cross talk, and influence each other, insulin sensitivity also improves at the liver and at the adipose tissue levels.

When resistance and aerobic exercise are undertaken in one exercise session, performing resistance exercise first results in less hypoglycemia than when aerobic exercise is performed first. Particularly, among those using insulin, or insulin providing therapies (medications that prod the beta cells to produce insulin).

It is important to remember though, an elderly person starting an exercise program after prolonged periods of inactivity must consult first with his doctor. That is being said, pre-exercise medical clearance is not necessary for most of asymptomatic individuals receiving diabetes care consistent with guidelines. That applies to those patients who wish to begin low- or moderate- intensity physical activity that is not exceeding the demands of brisk walking or everyday living.

Chapter 10

What if the Most Feared Thing Happens?

If and when diabetes is diagnosed, it comes with negative thoughts of all the possible complications. What is equally frightful is the belief that once a diabetic, will always be a diabetic.

However, over the last three decades, the more understanding and knowledge of diabetes as the outcome of increasing insulin resistance, and it's insidious evolvement at least in type 2 diabetes. The normal physiology of the insulin-secreting cells and other hormones has presented a new understanding, that many of the system failures can be reversible. After all, this disease may be curable.

That has been a dream for years and the goal of every scientist in the field.

More recently however, we have witnessed this dream come true, and diabetes cured, or rather, goes into a remission after bariatric surgery, often described as "metabolic" or "diabetes surgery."[31]

Truly, it will take drastic changes in weight and insulin sensitivity to put the diabetic state into a partial or total remission.

But still, it is a revolution, a breakthrough with hope and optimism for that to happen. At the very least, even those who experienced a relapse of their type 2 diabetes, after a period of remission, they experienced a drop in the rate of diabetic complications, specifically those, that affect the small blood vessels supplying the retinas, the kidneys, and the nerves.

In one study, for every one year free of diabetes, the risk of those complications dropped by 19 percent. The authors of the study called it "The legacy effect."[33]

The bottom line is this: weight loss works and insulin resistance, which is the culprit for the abnormal metabolic state, what we labeled as metabolic syndrome, can be reversed. In many instances, the reduction in meal sizes, and macronutrient composition brought down the insulin resistance and glucose levels even prior to the weight loss.

Now, in the previous chapter, I listed few general dietary guidelines regarding metabolic syndrome, its management, and ways to avoid progression to diabetes. Those general tips still hold for those diagnosed with diabetes. Here are some more specifics.

Because of the high energy of fat, the belief was, that increased dietary fat intake will lead to weight gain. So, the nutritional advice for obese individuals has often emphasized the avoidance of all types of dietary fat and their replacement with other macronutrients. In sharp contrast with this view, results from clinical trials testing low-fat diets for prevention of cardiovascular disease in postmenopausal women[34] and patients with diabetes[35] did not show any benefit of reduced fat intake in preventing heart disease.

Moreover, there was only marginal evidence of weight loss over time compared with normal diets. The results of a meta-analysis of trials comparing low-fat versus high-fat dietary interventions favored high-fat diets for weight loss, albeit, only in the context of calorie restriction.[36] In addition, long-term adherence to energy-restricted diets low in fat and high in complex carbohydrates to achieve weight loss is generally poor. Also, weight regain usually happens within six to twelve months after starting such diets.

The perception of dietary fat as unhealthy has resulted in decreased fat consumption in the United States over the past few decades. Yet both epidemics of obesity and diabetes have actually exploded.

Higher fat diets can be beneficial for the heart and blood vessels health if those fats come from non-animal sources. Ample evidence shows that the Mediterranean diet—a dietary pattern that includes high consumption of vegetable, and fish fats—is associated with lower all-cause mortality; that is deaths from all reasons including cardiovascular disease and cancer.[37]

The PREDIMED trial, conducted over five years among diabetics and nondiabetics, but with multiple risk factors for heart disease, compared two unrestricted-calorie Mediterranean diets—one enriched with extra-virgin olive oils and one with mixed nuts—and a control diet where the advice was to avoid all dietary fat.[38] A decrease in heart disease among individuals with type 2 diabetes was observed in those who followed the Mediterranean diets. At the end of the five-year study, the increase in waistline with aging was lower in the Mediterranean diets groups (less visceral fat) than in the control group. There was no weight gain in the two Mediterranean groups, and the group with the olive oil enrichment actually had weight loss.

Multiple explanations have been suggested, including the satiating effects of fat-rich foods, with ensuing displacement of other foods and sugary beverages that tend to increase visceral adiposity. Another is the positive, long-term effects of nuts, vegetables, and whole grains on adiposity and on lowering blood pressure. In addition, the modifying effect of the Mediterranean diet on our gut bacteria, what is termed *microbiota*, has been perceived as being positive by experts in the field.

Microbiota, as scientists are better in understanding its different populations and relation to diet, have been recently linked to the potential pathogenesis of multiple disease processes.

Oleic acid, which is a monounsaturated fatty acid and a primary component of olive oil, is a very common ingredient in the Mediterranean cuisine, and is reported to contribute to blood pressure lowering through an effect on cell membrane fluidity. It also lowers some of the adrenergic effects in our body, which is the heightened sympathetic activity, notably increased among insulin resistant individuals as previously explained.

Also MUFA- (monounsaturated fatty acids) rich foods like nuts, olive oil, and avocado contain numerous useful phenolic compounds, plants phyto-chemicals, and fat-soluble vitamins.

Many of those phenolic compounds are

protective against radical oxygen species. Radical oxygen species (ROS) are peroxides and free radicals that can inflict damage to the cell components, including base damage expressed as DNA strand breaks, and disruptions in cellular signaling.

The effect of ROS on our blood vessels, can be resembled by the effect of rust to metal pipes.

Medium chain triglycerides (MCT), whose fatty acids are Medium Chain Fatty Acids (MCFA) are also getting more recognition as a useful substitute of animal and saturated fat. To appreciate their value I will go back to the physiology of our body.

The human brain which is the largest of all other creatures brains considering the brain to the whole body size ratio, can utilize only glucose under normal conditions when food is available. When starvation is the case, the body glucose stores will be depleted in 5-6 days given that the brain alone consumes

125 grams daily, which is half the total body glucose consumption.

In the fasting state, as the insulin disappears, and glucagon is secreted, fat depots break their triglycerides into free fatty acids, those eventually reach the liver cells, and enter the mitochondria through a carnitine acyl transferase(CAT) system, which is a system of special enzymes. The body will then transform the fatty acids through a cycle of events into ketone bodies, like acetoacetate, and beta hydroxyl butyric acid (BHBA). The Ketone bodies and in particular BHBA will be utilized by the brain as a valuable alternate fuel, and now it can survive for another seventy days or so in case of starvation. Ketones and especially BHBA is an excellent fuel for the heart muscle as well.

Ketones tend to be an efficient fuel. Through the enhancement of the redox mechanism inside the mitochondria, not only do they generate and stack ATP efficiently which are energy storage packs, but also increase the mitochondrial defenses to fight radical oxygen species. Those oxide radicals as mentioned earlier play a significant role in illness, cellular damage and inflammation.[39]

Medium chain fatty acids (MCFA), those having 6-12 carbon atoms can enter the liver mitochondria independent of the CAT enzyme system, and become highly oxidized more than Long chain Fatty acids (LCFA) which are 16-18 carbons long. MCFA can generate ketone bodies within the mitochondria much easier than their longer chain peers. The MCFA aqueous solubility facilitates their easy penetration through the double mitochondrial membranes and their quick incorporation into Krebs cycle. That makes them specially equipped in producing ketones, the highly efficient power units much needed in times of stress.

Their ability to make ketones easier is an advantage when more efficient energy sources are needed. As when glucose and other energy sources are harder to attain, either because of a shortage, or compromised delivery. Recent data with newer diabetes drugs that favored ketones accumulation, like Empagliflozin, as I will elaborate later, showed better heart and kidneys function, and reduced the incidence of heart failure significantly.

MCFA, as they have more aqueous solubility, they do not need to be emulsified and hydrolyzed as LCFA. And being easily absorbed through enterocytes of the intestine, they do not need to be packaged as chylomicrons, or to go through lymphatics and eventually to the systemic circulation. So the post-prandial (after a meal) spike in triglycerides is minimal or absent. Instead they are easily absorbed into the portal circulation, and to the liver.

This is especially valuable in patients with severe hypertriglyceridemia, where their own natural mechanisms to clear chylomicrons, and hydrolyze their triglyceride load are disabled.

MCFA are also lesser calorie dense. They have 8.3 calories per gram versus 9 calories per gram in case of the regular fat.

They tend to be more utilized, stored less, and accordingly less likely to be ectopically (where they do not belong) stored. Their enhanced metabolism has been shown in the form of higher post-prandial thermogenesis (more of the meal is spent in the form of heat generation) in human studies.

Few studies reported improvement in insulin sensitivity when MCFA sources comprised at least 24 percent of the total daily calories provided.

Given the fact that calorie-restricted diets are often associated with marked decline in energy expenditure, foods rich in MCFA can improve the long term success of dietary management of obesity by spiking the energy expenditure instead.[40]

MCT represent about 10-20% of the fat content of cow, goat, and sheep milk. Coconut oil has about 50% of its total fat in the form of MCT. It sounds like an excellent alternative to conventional fat sources.

Equally important to the quality and nutrient composition of the meals is the quantity: serving sizes and number of helpings.

Scientific data warns of large fluctuations in blood glucose levels. Those fluctuations can hurt the blood vessels. The more the fluctuations, in both magnitude and frequency, the more is the generation of super-oxide radicals that can cause damage to the endothelial cells that line the arteries and arterioles.

A prominent scientist once stated, "We are as old as our arteries." This is why doctors stress the importance, for diabetics, of smaller and more frequent meals.

This should be the norm rather than

the exception. The smaller meals lower those risky fluctuations in the blood sugars particularly after meals. This is doubly important when Diabetes treatment includes insulin or medications that increase the release of insulin. Higher blood glucose levels require higher doses of insulin. Then the patient's glucose goes from high to low, triggering a pattern of defensive eating, and so go high again. The patients get caught in this roller coaster, and in addition to gaining more weight from the defensive eating, the real victim of those glycemic fluctuations are the arteries. Our goal is to protect those arteries. They are the conduits of life, and whenever blocked, illness and death is not far behind.

So the state of the arteries, determines this semi-medical description known as the "biological age". Older individuals who took care of their health (combined with the privilege of good genes), while chronologically are in their eighties, may have a biological age of mid or early sixty because of their arteries health, and the reverse is also true.

Chapter 11

Medications we use for treating Diabetes

The discovery of insulin was a lifesaving breakthrough. It is a replacement of a hormone that is missing as in type 1 diabetes. In type 2 diabetes, insulin became so ineffective and insufficient in the face of an increasing insulin resistance, that more of it is needed from external sources.

Insulins have improved with technological advances, basal insulins tend to be longer acting and peak-less, to copy normal physiology of basal slowly pulsatile insulin secretion. Short acting or prandial insulin, became shorter over the years, quicker in action to try to imitate the physiological spike of insulin with meals, without lingering around after the meal induced glucose spike abates. This is a way designed to avoid glucose fluctuations, and minimize the defensive eating and weight gain seen universally with insulin treatment.

Early on, after the introduction of insulin, came the sulphonylureas, a family of drugs that work to prod the beta cells to make more insulin, even though they were tired, overworked, and almost burned out. That is why those oral medications will lose their efficacy over the years, the beta cells simply collapse, and flogging disabled horses does not work. Besides, as those drugs increase insulin secretion, low blood glucose levels, and accordingly defensive eating is a common scenario, and weight gain is a common side effect of those drugs as well. Those medications while very effective are losing favor among diabetes specialists for the previously listed reasons.

As the knowledge of insulin resistance evolved over the last several decades, a search for medications that can offset the insulin resistance, and restore back the sensitivity of the body tissues to insulin, became the theme of diabetes research.

Metformin, a drug extracted from a natural flower, became soon a favorite, either by itself or in combination with other drugs. It helps the liver to shut up when it was not needed to pour more glucose. It also works on the gut to form more incretins like GLP1. As mentioned earlier, GLP1 facilitate insulin release in proportion to the work load. That is to say in proportion to the glucose level, making low blood sugar, and thus overeating less likely. The latter is very valuable in avoiding weight gain.

Then came another family of drugs, called thiazolidinediones, one popular member is pioglitazone. Those are a fascinating group of drugs that work on special receptors in the nucleus of the cell. They reprogram the cellular signaling, and end up making more fat cells. While that makes little sense, why creating more fat cells when there are plenty?

If the reader remembers earlier what I mentioned about fatty acids.

Fatty acids are loose cannons, showering the liver, the skeletal muscles, the beta cells, and even the heart muscles.

The newly formed healthy fat cells formed by the pioglitazone and other thiazolidinediones, will contain and confine those loose cannons. So the beta cells will rid itself of those fatty acids, and be able to recover slowly and gradually, as the toxic effect or lipotoxicity of those fatty acids resolves.

The skeletal muscles lose those fats as well, and they turn to become more insulin sensitive, the liver similarly getting rid of the depositing fat, becomes insulin sensitive as well.

The total subcutaneous fat cells increase with pioglitazone about 4 %, while the visceral adipose tissue, the ectopic fat is reduced by about 20 %. That is to say, it restores back the natural metabolic sinks, the subcutaneous fat, while cutting out ectopic fat sites.

Recent studies revealed reduction in cardiovascular disease with the pioglitazone, as well as preventing the progression of pre-diabetics to frank diabetes as shown in the IRIS trial.[41]

Then incretins, like GLP1 were later on introduced. Those are GLP1 similar molecules, that can bind to the GLP1 receptors in the body and mimic the action of that valuable hormone that tend to be gravely diminished in type 2 diabetic patients. Drugs like Exenetide, liraglutide, lixisenetide, and semaglutide are examples of the GLP1 receptor agonists (working on receptors to activate them like the natural GLP1 hormone).

Those agents, called at times incretin mimetics (as they imitate the naturally secreted incretin hormone) proved very useful in lowering glucose while reducing the body weight, as they restore insulin sensitivity, curb the appetite and slow the gastric (Stomach) emptying. Some of those injectable agents are given daily, some weekly, and research is ongoing to soon provide monthly administered agents. Again recent studies showed reduction in cardiovascular events like heart attacks with those agents, as revealed in the Leader trial with liraglutide. A big advantage those drugs added is the reduced blood glucose fluctuations specifically after meals.[42]

Almost simultaneously, another family of drugs, named DPP4 inhibitors, was introduced. Simply, those agents deactivate the enzyme that breaks down the natural

GLP1, so the little that is there survive enough to add up to some more, and so on, until reaching a critical mass to be effective again. The enzyme DPP4 (Dipeptidyl peptidase 4) makes the GLP1 survive for few minutes, when deactivated, the GLP1 survive for hours instead. Again they lower glucose without increasing the body weight, a common adverse effect we see with insulin and sulphonylureas.

More recently, a family of glucoretics was introduced, as the name implies, simply making the diabetics urinate out the glucose building up in their blood stream.

Those agents are named SGLT2 inhibitors since they inhibit or block a group of transporting proteins named SGLT2 (sodium-glucose transporters type 2) in the kidneys proximal tubules.

Those transporters, under normal conditions help the kidneys to absorb back any glucose leaking in the urine, a self-preservation instinct to keep the glucose from being wasted, even though there is plenty of it in the case of diabetes.

As those agents block those transporters, glucose topping above 100 mg/dl will start leaking in the urine. Patients tend to urinate excessively until the glucose in the blood is lowered significantly.

As diabetics lose glucose in the urine, those wasted calories translate into weight loss, provided that the patients adapt also a healthier life style as I pointed earlier in the book.

Recent studies again showed significant reduction in cardiovascular disease with those SGLT2 inhibitors, the studied drug was empagliflozin, and the study name was empa-reg trial.[43]

Conclusion

In closing, I hope I succeeded to make my case, explaining why and how our eating and activity styles can be our worse enemies. And how our visceral adipocytes can be deadly in sabotaging the normal physiological harmony designed in our magnificently engineered bodies.

If you came away with an understanding of what is normal and what went wrong, then I am very optimistic you can start acting now to change your path. Choose a balanced diet you like, using some guiding tips that I suggested earlier, and the type of exercise activity you enjoy the most.

By recognizing the signs and symptoms

that we or our loved ones have of that metabolic syndrome, we may be able to reduce the risk of losing the natural elasticity of the arteries. By preventing them from becoming rigid and sick, we might be able to prevent heart attacks and strokes.

The most recognizable feature of metabolic syndrome is a big waistline; more than 94 cm in men and more than 80 cm in women. This is true for most ethnic groups. The second feature is a triglyceride level above 150 mg/dl. The third one is high blood pressure, equal or above 130/85 in the absence of blood pressure medications, or lower in presence of blood pressure medications.

The fourth feature is a low HDL cholesterol; below 50 mg/dl in women and below 40 mg/dl in men.

A fifth criterion is high fasting blood glucose, above 100 mg/dl. It still can be below 126 in nondiabetics; 126 and higher in those with diabetes.

It takes only three of those factors to make the diagnosis of metabolic syndrome, but as they add up, the risk grows higher and higher for the blood vessels to become gradually and progressively more rigid, thus increasing the risk for heart attacks and strokes.

It is not a secret that cardiovascular disease is the number one killer for both men and women in the civilized world. Knowledge is power, but only if it leads to action. And that is what I am hoping for.

The goal, I hope that this book will accomplish, is to equip every reader with insightful prudence. Learning what is the normal and what went wrong, or better still what can go wrong, is a platform for better understanding. From that point on, an intentional change for a better health is the desired fruit.

Take small and consistent steps that add up over time to real milestones. May be you should start eating a good healthy breakfast, fortified with good proteins that can sustain you longer. And avoid skipping meals, something that for sure will set you up for hunger and oversized portions later in the day when you are more likely to be tired and less active.

Do not wait until starving to eat, you are going to overdo it, and then regret it. The more guilt, the faster people give up. Build gradually physical activity into your daily schedule. Increments of ten minutes three or four times a day will add up, and are easier to come by than a dedicated thirty to forty five minutes.

Try something fun, you do not have to run. Try a mix of aerobic and resistance activities, and build a routine of your favorites in your own sequence. You build it, stick with it, and be patient. Swallowing a pill sometimes may sound easier than swallowing the logic of a balanced life style. Believe me, after many years of treating patients, pills alone do not work. It takes commitment and choices to make for pills to work, so why not do it before needing the pill.

However, my input is by no means a replacement of your doctor's advice. Think of it as an extension of an education chance, a closer look into the body remarkable engineering. Respecting the beauty of our body structure and function, is an initial step to take better care of it.

Notes

1   M. I. Harris, R. Klein, T. A. Welborn, and M. W. Knuiman, "Onset of NIDDM Occurs at Least 4-7 Years Before Clinical Diagnosis," *Diabetes Care* 15 (1992): 815–19.

2   E. M. Wright, B. A. Hirayama, and D. F. Loo, "Active Sugar Transport in Health and Disease," *Journal of internal Medicine* 261 (2007): 32-43.

3   P. Rorsman, L. Eliasson, E. Renstrom, J. Gromada, S. Barg, and S. Gopel, "The Cell Physiology of Biphasic Insulin Secretion," *News in Physiological Sciences : An International Journal of Physiology, produced jointly by the International Union of Physiological Sciences and the American Physiological Society* 15 (2000): 72–77.

4   R. J. Schulingkamp, T. C. Pagano, D. Hung, and R. B. Raffa, "Insulin Receptors and Insulin Action in the Brain: Review and Clinical Implications," *Neuroscience and Biobehavioral Reviews* 24 (2000): 855–72.

5   R. A. DeFronzo and D. Tripathy, "Skeletal Muscle Insulin Resistance is the Primary Defect in Type 2 Diabetes," *Diabetes Care* 32 Suppl 2 (2009):S157–63.

6   J. Lindstrom, P. Ilanne-Parikka, M. Peltonen, et al., "Sustained Reduction in the Incidence of Type 2 Diabetes by Lifestyle Intervention: Follow-up of the Finnish Diabetes Prevention Study. *Lancet* 368 (2006): 1673–679.

7   S. Basu, M. McKee, G. Galea, and D. Stuckler, "Relationship of Soft Drink Consumption to Global Overweight, Obesity, and Diabetes: A Cross-national Analysis of 75 Countries," *American Journal of Public Health* 103 (2013): 2071–77.

8   A. Kotronen, L. Juurinen, M. Tiikkainen, S. Vehkavaara, and H. Yki-Jarvinen, "Increased Liver Fat, Impaired Insulin Clearance, and Hepatic and Ddipose Tissue Insulin Resistance in Type 2 diabetes," *Gastroenterology* 135 (2008): 122–30.

9   A. Tcherno and J. P. Despres, "Pathophysiology of Human Visceral Obesity: An Update," *Physiological Reviews* 93 (2013): 359–404.

10 Y. Wang, E. B. Rimm, M. J. Stampfer, H. C. Willett, and F. B. Hu, "Comparison of Abdominal

Adiposity and Overall Obesity in Predicting Risk of Type 2 Diabetes Among Men.," The American Journal of Clinical Nutrition 81 (2005): 555–63.

[11] V. R. Soman, V. A. Koivisto, D. Deibert, P. Felig, and R. A. DeFronzo, "Increased Insulin Sensitivity and Insulin Binding to Monocytes After Physical Training," *New England Journal of Medicine* 301 (1979): 1200–4.

[12] Y. Nishida, K. Tokuyama, S. Nagasaka, et al., "Effect of Moderate Exercise Training on Peripheral Glucose Effectiveness, Insulin Sensitivity, and Endogenous Glucose Production in Healthy Humans Estimated by a Two-Compartment-Labeled Minimal Model," *Diabetes* 53 (2004): 315–20.

[13] G. Jiang and B. B. Zhang, "Glucagon and Regulation of Glucose Metabolism," *American Journal of Physiology Endocrinology and Metabolism* 284 (2003):E671–78.

[14] S. S. Hammerstad, S. F. Grock, H. J. Lee, A. Hasham, N. Sundaram, and Y. Tomer, "Diabetes and Hepatitis C: A Two-Way Association," *Frontiers in Endocrinology* 6 (2015): 134.

[15] D. J. Drucker and M. A. Nauck, "The Incretin System: Glucagon-like Peptide-1 Receptor

Agonists and Dipeptidyl Peptidase-4 Inhibitors in Type 2 Diabetes. *Lancet* 368 (2006): 1696–705.

16 D. J. Drucker and M. A. Nauck, "The Incretin System: Glucagon-like Peptide-1 Receptor Agonists and Dipeptidyl Peptidase-4 Inhibitors in Type 2 Diabetes. *Lancet* 368 (2006): 1696–705.

17 T. A. Lutz, "Effects of Amylin on Eating and Adiposity," *Handbook of Experimental Pharmacology* (2012) :231–50.

18 "Postprandial Blood Glucose," American Diabetes Association. *Diabetes Care* 24 (2001): 775–78.

19 J. M. Wojcicki and M. B. Heyman, "Let's Move—Childhood Obesity Prevention from Pregnancy and Infancy Onward," *New England Journal of Medicine* 362 (2010): 1457–459.

20 J. P. Despres, B. Lamarche, P. Mauriege, et al., "Hyperinsulinemia as an Independent Risk Factor for Ischemic Heart Disease," *New England Journal of Medicine* 334 (1996): 952–57.

21 J. T. Salonen, T. A. Lakka, H. M., Lakka, V. P. Valkonen, S. A. Everson, and G. A. Kaplan, "Hyperinsulinemia Is Associated With the Incidence of Hypertension and Dyslipidemia in Middle-Aged Men," *Diabetes* 47 (1998): 270–75.

22 "Appropriate Body-Mass Index for Asian Populations and Its Implications for Policy

and Intervention Strategies, *Lancet* 363 (2004):157–63.

23 C. J. Fielding and P. E. Fielding, "Cholesterol Transport Between Cells and Body Fluids: Role of Plasma Lipoproteins and the Plasma Cholesterol Esterification System," *Medical Clinics of North America* 66 (1982): 363–73.

24 W. C. Cromwell and J. D. Otvos, "Heterogeneity of Low-Density Lipoprotein Particle Number in Patients With Type 2 Diabetes Mellitus and Low-Density Lipoprotein Cholesterol <100 mg/dl," *American Journal of Cardiology* 98 (2006): 1599–602.

25 R. L. Koffarnus, L. M. Mican, D. A. Lopez, and J. C. Barner, "Evaluation of an Inpatient Psychiatric Hospital Physician Education Program and Adherence to American Diabetes Association Practice Recommendations," *American Journal of Health-System Pharmacy: AJHP, Official Journal of the American Society of Health-System Pharmacists* 73 (2016):S57–62.

26 E. M. Koehler, J. N. Schouten, B. E. Hansen, et al., "Prevalence and Risk Factors of Non-alcoholic Fatty Liver Disease in the Elderly: Results from the Rotterdam Study," *Journal of Hepatology* 57 (2012): 1305–11.

27 K. L. Stanhope, J. M. Schwarz, N. L. Keim, et al., "Consuming Fructose-Sweetened, Not Glucose-Sweetened Beverages Increases Visceral Adiposity and Lipids and Decreases Insulin Sensitivity in Overweight/Obese Humans. *Journal of Clinical Investigation* 119 (2009): 1322–334.

28 H. E. Bays, P. H. Jones, C. E. Orringer, W. V. Brown, and T. A. Jacobson TA. "National Lipid Association Annual Summary of Clinical Lipidology 2016," *Journal of Clinical Lipidology* 10 (2016): S1–43.

29 M. Boschmann, J. Steiniger, U. Hille, et al., "Water-Induced Thermogenesis," *The Journal of Clinical Endocrinology and Metabolism* 88 (2003): 6015–6019.

30 P. T. Katzmarzyk, T. S. Church, C. L. Craig, and C. Bouchard, "Sitting Time and Mortality From All Causes, Cardiovascular Disease, and Cancer," *Medicine and Science in Sports and Exercise* 41 (2009): 998–1005.

31 H. Buchwald, R. Estok, K. Fahrbach, et al., "Weight and Type 2 Diabetes After Bariatric Surgery: Systematic Review and Meta-analysis," *American Journal of Medicine* 122 (2009): 248–56, e5.

32 V. L. Gloy, M. Briel, D. L. Bhatt, et al., "Bariatric Surgery Versus Non-surgical Treatment for Obesity: A Systematic Review and Meta-analysis of Randomised Controlled trials," *BMJ* (Clinical research ed) 347 (2013): f5934.

33 K. J. Coleman, S. Haneuse, E. Johnson, et al., "Long-Term Microvascular Disease Outcomes in Patients With Type 2 Diabetes After Bariatric Surgery: Evidence for the Legacy Effect of Surgery," *Diabetes Care* 39 (2016): 1400–7.

34 B. V. Howard B, L. Van Horn, J. Hsia, et al., "Low-Fat Dietary Pattern and Risk of Cardiovascular Disease: The Women's Health Initiative Randomized Controlled Dietary Modification Trial," *Journal of American Medicine* 295 (2006): 655–66.

35 R. R. Wing, P. Bolin, F. L. Brancati, et al., "Cardiovascular Effects of Intensive Lifestyle Intervention in Type 2 Diabetes," *New England Journal of Medicine* 369 (2013): 145–54.

36 D. K. Tobias, M. Chen, J. E. Manson, D. S. Ludwig, W. Willett, and F. B. Hu, "Effect of Low-Fat Diet Interventions Versus Other Diet Interventions on Long-Term Weight Change in Adults: A Systematic Review and Meta-analysis. *The Lancet Diabetes & Endocrinology* 3 (2015): 968–79.

37   F. Sofi, R. Abbate, G. F. Gensini, and A. Casini, "Accruing Evidence on Benefits of Adherence to the Mediterranean Diet on Health: An Updated Systematic Review and Meta-analysis. The American Journal of Clinical Nutrition 92 (2010): 1189–96.

38   R. Estruch, E. Ros, J. Salas-Salvado, et al., "Primary Prevention of Cardiovascular Disease With a Mediterranean Diet. New England Journal of Medicine 368 (2013): 1279–90.

39   D. Ward, "MCT Beneficial Effects on Energy, Atherosclerosis and Aging," *Nutrition Review* (2013).

40   S.A. Rial, A.D. Karelis, et al., K.F. Bergeron, et al., "Gut Microbiota and Metabolic Health. The potential Beneficial Effects of a Medium Chain Triglyceride Diet in Obese Individuals." *Nutrients* 8.5 (2016): 281.

41   S.E. Inzucchi, C.M. Viscoli, and L.H. Young, "Pioglitazone Prevents Diabetes in Patients With Insulin Resistance and Cerebrovascular Disease." *Diabetes Care* 39.10 (2016): 1684-1692.

42   S.P. Marso, G.H. Daniels, K. Brown-Frandsen, et al., "Liraglutide and cardiovascular outcomes in type 2 diabetes." *New England Journal of Medicine* 375.4 (2016): 311-322.

[43] B. Zinman, C. Wanner, J.M. Lachin, et al., "Empagliflozin, cardiovascular outcomes, and mortality in type 2 diabetes." *New England Journal of Medicine* 373.22 (2015): 2117-2128.